# WHEAT FREE KID?!?

# NOW WHAT?

A GUIDE TO HELP YOU ON YOUR JOURNEY FROM A MOM WHO HAS BEEN THERE

# Wheat free?  This cannot be happening to me! What in the world will I feed this child?

Chances are if you have downloaded this booklet, you are in great need of advice, compassion, and ideas to help you muddle through this issue.  I am here to tell you that I know exactly where you're coming from.  I remember hearing the diagnosis from the doctor telling me that my six year old son was allergic to wheat and should be on a wheat free diet.  The panic set in immediately.  Oh, no, I thought, he's going to starve.  I don't know what to feed this kid.  What am I going to do?

Lucky for you this world has come a long way since 2002.  When I began on this abyss of wheat free food, there was very little information or product out there for a kid like mine.  Now it is different.  Now you have a myriad of choices and I hope that this little book will get you off on the right path without the pain of buying a boat load of products that even your dog wouldn't eat.

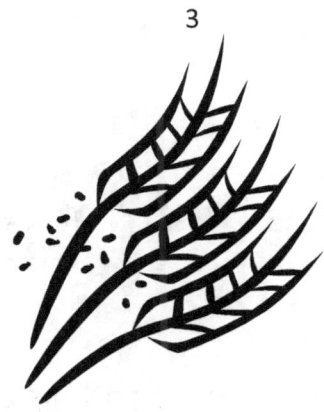

Welcome to the Wheat Free World!!

It is an easy world now, I assure you. Make sure that your child is indeed wheat sensitive. By this I mean that when he/she ingests any wheat product, they feel sick, bloated, have gas, diarrhea, abdominal pain, or any feeling of "Oh, why did I eat that?" Some kids are truly allergic which means they break out in hives, can't breathe, and itch all over. Wheat sensitivity and wheat allergy are two different things. But I have a hunch they both can be solved and managed in a Wheat Free World.

Here's the first thing you need to know: Eating absolutely no wheat is very possible. I bet you won't even miss it. Wheat is hard to digest for a lot of people and there are plenty of alternatives to it. Without beating around the bush let's get to the nitty gritty of changing your child's diet:

# 1. Substitute rice flour for regular flour:

- Find it in the natural food aisle of any large grocery store or order it online: I like Bob's Red Mill Rice Flour. It comes in a larger than usual package and can be directly substituted for any recipe calling for flour.
- It tastes very light and fluffy when mixed with baking powder. All of my kids devour the rice flour pancakes I make. (I never even told them what the difference was-they just love them)
- Bake, bake bake. I know, I know, it takes time but it is worth it. It tastes good and saves you money. The wheat free and gluten free cookies at the store cost a lot and they don't taste that great. Your cookies will taste better and your child will never forget what you're doing for him/her.
- Buy ready made things when you have to. I know I just said bake, but sometimes you need the convenience more than the taste. Go easy on yourself-you're a good parent!

## 2. Buy digestive enzymes.

- Plant based digestive enzymes can be purchased at any vitamin store. Giving one before every meal has helped my son with feeling uncomfortable fullness after he eats.
- If your child is only wheat sensitive, you could even try the enzymes and see if that remedies the issue.

- They're perfectly safe and not expensive. They simply aid in digestion so your child's body doesn't work so hard to digest nutrients he/she needs.

## 3. Buy rice pasta

- I love the Tinkyada brand. It is just so good and does not get mushy when you boil it. I make it all the time for my kids and they ask for it even though the other three are not wheat sensitive. You can make it with mozzarella, sauce, parmesan, tuna, as mac and cheese. The options are the same as regular pasta.

4. **Rice cakes instead of bread.**

- Does this sound gross to you?  Just take my word for it and try it.  The Quaker brand rice cakes are light and kind of taste like popcorn.  I spread peanut butter and jelly on one and top it with another.  It really is tasty and very portable. The reason I suggest this is because bread made from rice flour did not work for us; not only the cost, but the taste.  I suggest rice cakes as an alternative to you for lunches, snacks, etc.  Perhaps you can get your hands on a bread recipe that uses rice flour and is tasty-I haven't found one yet and I've wasted a lot of money and energy trying everything I could get my hands on.

5. **Spelt Bread**

- Spelt is an ancient grain from the Middle East and has different properties than wheat.  Some people who can't handle wheat can digest spelt.  I used this initially when my son was little because I could toast it and put his favorite peanut butter and jelly on it.  It looked familiar to him and he would eat it.  The cost is high, however, but you can order it online from Berlin Natural Bakery in Ohio.  Amish people make it and will ship it to your home.  Like I mentioned, the cost is high but it is an option if you don't mind spending more.

## 6. Fruits and Vegetables

- Being wheat sensitive usually means that the stomach is not happy with processed and fatty foods. We all love the taste of McDonald's fries but when they hit a wheat sensitive tummy it is not worth the pain. I have found that fruit helps my son's stomach feel better. I don't claim to be a doctor but the naturally occurring fiber in apples, peaches, pears, and nectarines have helped my son's tummy calm down and quiet down. We all hear the mantra of fruits and veges are the best way to stay healthy and maintain a healthy weight. That's true. But they can also calm down a disturbed stomach.

# MEAL IDEAS THAT TAKE OUT THE GUESSWORK:

## Breakfast:

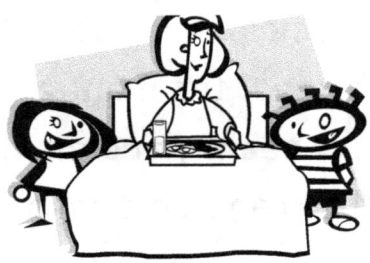

- ✓ Oatmeal with brown sugar
- ✓ Rice flour pancakes with butter and syrup
- ✓ Rice flour pancakes with turkey sausage
- ✓ Corn Flakes
- ✓ Frosted Flakes
- ✓ Captain Crunch cereal
- ✓ Honey Nut Corn Flakes
- ✓ Muffins made with rice flour

Rice Dream beverage is great on cereals-

## Mom's Gluten Free Pancakes

| | |
|---|---|
| 1 cup rice flour | 1 egg |
| ½ tsp baking powder | Chocolate chips (optional) |
| ½ tsp salt | |
| ¼ cup vegetable oil | |
| ½ cup milk | |

Preheat a skillet over medium heat. Combine dry ingredients in a mixing bowl. Add oil, egg, and milk with a whisk. Combine until most of the lumps are out. On the hot skillet pour the batter in circles. Add chocolate chips if desired and flip with a spatula when bubbles are in the center. Allow the other side of the pancake to cook and remove to serving plate. Makes 4-6 pancakes depending on the size. Serve hot with butter and syrup.

# LUNCH:

- ✓ **Rice cakes with choice of toppings**: peanut butter and jelly, tuna salad, egg salad, chicken salad
- ✓ **Toasted spelt bread made the way they like it.**
- ✓ **Peanut butter and banana slices**
- ✓ **Peanut butter and celery sticks**
- ✓ **Apples with caramel sauce for dipping**
- ✓ **Rice noodles with sauce and cheese**
- ✓ **Grilled cheese made with spelt/rice bread**-sometimes when this type of bread is toasted or grilled it tastes a lot better

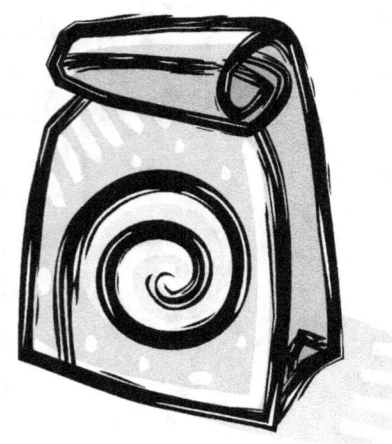

# Try this:

**Brown Bag Lunch**

2 rice cakes-any flavor

1 Tbs peanut butter

1 Tbs jelly

Bag of chips

Cut up fruit

Beverage

Spread the peanut butter and jelly on one cake and top with the other. Assemble the rest of the lunch contents and pop them all in a brown bag. It is so easy, you'll wonder why you didn't think of it before.

# DINNER:

- ✓ **Side dish of rice pasta**
- ✓ **Side dish of any potato**
- ✓ **Side dish of any type of rice**
- ✓ **Vegetables with salt and cheese**
- ✓ **Meat choices are limitless**
- ✓ **Sliced fruit in a bowl-**I love to throw a bowl of orange slices on the table at dinner time. They help themselves and I've managed to get another serving of fruit in them.

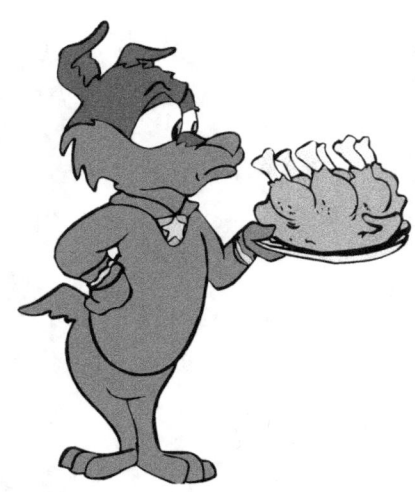

# A WORD ABOUT MEAT:

**Meat is important to a growing body. I realize that there are vegans out there that do not eat meat and that is fine. For the rest of us, this can be a hard choice due to the nature of factory farming. Please consider these options:**

*Organic hot dogs –* Consider this instead of your major brand of hot dogs. There are brands that do not use any fillers, nitrates, or artificial ingredients. Also, all of the animals used for these foods are grass fed and treated humanely-believe me-it makes for a great tasting hot dog. You can get gluten free hot dog buns but they tend to fall apart. We just eat our hot dogs plain or dip them in ketchup. I even cut them up and mix them with veges and rice noodles. If that doesn't sound too appetizing, experiment with what your family prefers.

*Organic beef and chicken -* There is a difference between regular meat you buy at the store and organic meat. Organic meat means that the cattle are fed grass and the chickens are allowed to roam. The animals are healthier for it and it comes out in the taste. I'm not a PETA member but treating animals humanely is important to me and my kids. Your conscience can be clear when your family has organic meat for dinner. Also, there are no grain fillers in this type of meat. No chance of a hidden tummy ache. We buy from a local farmer but more and more stores have a small selection of organic beef and chicken. Make sure it is organic and not just "natural". If the label does not emphasize grass fed cattle or free range chickens it is not organic. A good brand is Applegate Farms.

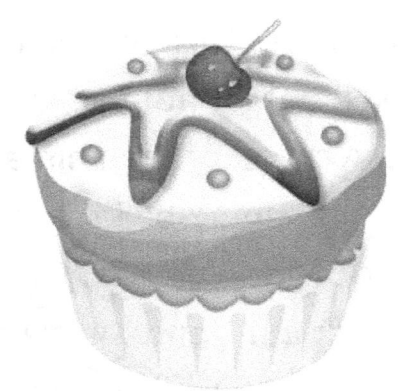

## DESSERTS AND BAKED GOODS

Yum. Nothing like a piece of chocolate cake or a rich brownie to chow on. Don't fret-there are so many great mixes out there you'll have to exercise the will power not to eat all of them! Pamela's Products is a great source of cake mixes, brownie mixes, and cookie mixes that are all gluten free. The brownie mix is our favorite-they are hands down the best I have ever tasted. I buy the mixes at the store and they are pricey but for a special occasion or a nice treat they are a stress free option. The directions are on the bag and they're easy as can be.

# Mom's Best Chocolate Chip Cookies

| | |
|---|---|
| 2 sticks of butter | 1 tsp vanilla |
| ½ cup sugar | 2 cups rice flour |
| ½ cup brown sugar | 1 tsp baking soda |
| 2 eggs | ½ tsp salt |

Preheat the oven to 350 degrees.  Mix the butter and both sugars in a large mixing bowl, scraping the sides until well blended.  Add the eggs one at a time being sure to scrape down the bowl until well blended.  Add the vanilla and continue to mix.  Add one cup of flour at a time on a slow speed.  Add the baking soda and salt while the mixer is moving.  If you prefer a denser cookie, add an additional ½ cup rice flour until you achieve the desired consistency.

Drop dough on an ungreased cookie sheet and bake for 7-9 minutes.  Remove and cool on a wire rack.  Yield: 2 dozen cookies.  Store in an airtight container in the refrigerator.

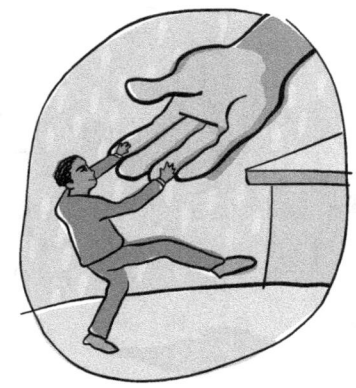

## A Word of Encouragement:

I think this is a good time to mention that just because one person has a food allergy in your family doesn't mean that person has to be isolated from good food. Having this allergy issue may make all of you eating better and healthier. This economy we're in doesn't make it easy to manage a food allergy but it can be done if you're armed with information before you spend the money at the store. I cannot tell you how much money I have spent on foods that were downright nasty. Please remember that planning ahead of time makes for less spending once you're at the store because you're not in a panic.

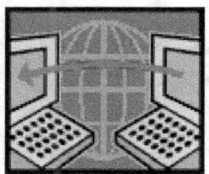

If your local store doesn't carry gluten free foods, try the websites. Here are some that I have used time and time again:

www.tinkyada.com

www.applegatefarms.com

www.berlinnaturalbakery.com

www.wallacefarms.com They have buying clubs in the Midwest region

www.pamelasproducts.com


I'm sure there are more to choose from depending on where you live. Hop on the web and see what you can find.

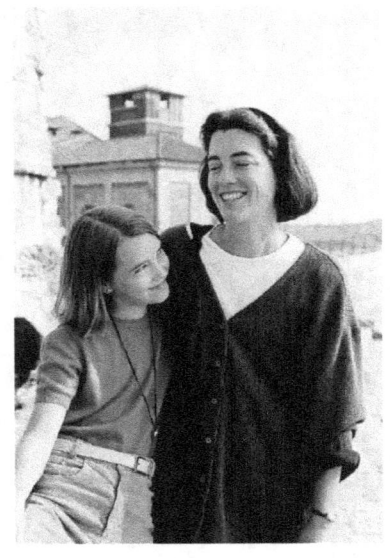

Remember, this is a manageable issue. Your love for your child will propel you to change what needs to be changed. If you're feeling overwhelmed, just re-read the lists I give in this booklet and stick to it until your confidence is up and you can branch out in other directions. If something I have suggested is not for you, don't worry about it. These are descriptions, not prescriptions. You know your child best and you will make the right choices for him/her!

# Price Lists:

Approximate Costs as of publishing:

Bob's Red Mill Rice Flour         $5.00/2 lb bag

Bob's Red Mill Pancake Mix    $5.00/1 lb bag

Pamela's Brownie Mix             $6.50/bag

Pamela's Chocolate Cake Mix  $6.50/bag

Blueberry Muffin recipe:          $7.50/2 dozen home made

Chocolate Chip Cookies:         $6.00/2 dozen home made

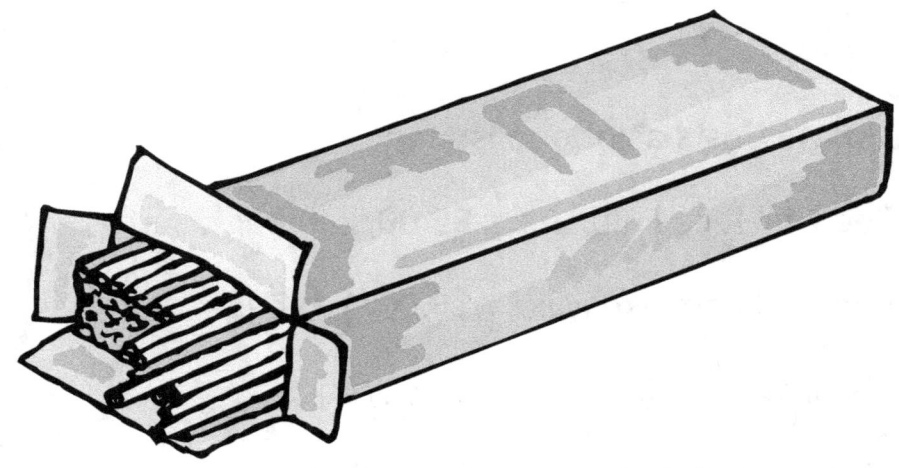

## The Best Noodles Ever

1 package Tinkyada rice noodles, any shape

3 cups boiling water

1 Tbs sea salt

Barilla Garden Vegetable Spaghetti Sauce

¼ cup grated parmesan cheese


Prepare the rice noodles according to package directions

Drain when at desired consistency and place in serving bowl.  Pour the sauce over the noodles and mix.  Top with the parmesan cheese-Dinner is served!


You can use any type of cheese with this recipe.

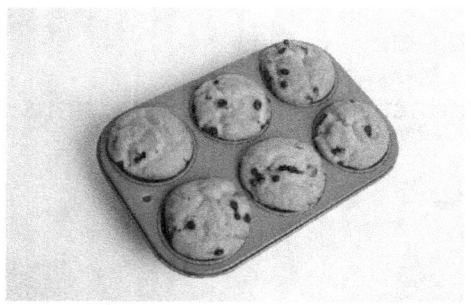

# Blueberry Muffins

1 ½ cup rice flour

½  tsp baking soda

½ tsp salt

¾ cup of sugar

½ cup (1 stick) of butter

2 large eggs

½ cup blueberry yogurt

½ cup fresh blueberries

¼ cup rice milk or cow milk

1 tsp vanilla extract

Preheat the oven to 375 degrees.  Place muffin liners in two muffin pans.  Combine the dry ingredients in a small mixing bowl.  In a large bowl, cream together the butter and sugar.  Beat in the eggs one at a time.  Add the yogurt, milk, and vanilla; mix until smooth.  Stir in the dry mixture just until moistened.  Stir in the blueberries.

Spoon the batter into the prepared muffin liners.  Bake for 15-20 minutes or until fork ready. Be sure to watch them carefully as the rice flour is more delicate than regular flour. Yield 24 muffins.

Please feel free to contact me with any questions, comments or concerns:

mihicshouse@comcast.net

Thank you for reading this booklet.

I truly pray that it takes the guess work out of your child's health issue. Knowledge is power and eliminates the panic button!

Thanks!

Jennifer Mihic

**PERSONAL REFLECTIONS:**

**PERSONAL REFLECTIONS:**

www.ingramcontent.com/pod-product-compliance
Lightning Source LLC
Chambersburg PA
CBHW081813280526
45789CB00008B/3115